The
NEW USMLE
Step 2 CS

101 Myths Debunked

The
NEW USMLE
Step 2 CS

101 Myths Debunked

Brenda R. Affinati, MD, FACP

Associate Program Director of Internal Medicine
Department of Internal Medicine
Advocate Lutheran General Hospital
Park Ridge, Illinois
Associate Professor of Medicine
Department of Medicine
Chicago Medical School Rosalind Franklin
University of Medicine and Science
North Chicago, Illinois

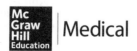

New York / Chicago / San Francisco / Athens / London / Madrid
Mexico City / Milan / New Delhi / Singapore / Sydney / Toronto

The New USMLE Step 2 CS: 101 Myths Debunked

1 2 3 4 5 6 7 8 9 0   DOC/DOC   18 17 16 15 14 13

ISBN 978-0-07-182813-0
MHID 0-07-182813-3

This book was set in Minion Pro by Thomson Digital.
The editors were Catherine A. Johnson and Cindy Yoo.
The production supervisor was Catherine Saggese.
Project management was provided by Ritu Joon, Thomson Digital.
RR Donnelley was printer and binder.

This book is printed on acid-free paper.

Library of Congress Cataloging-in-Publication Data

Affinati, Brenda R., author.
  The new USMLE step 2 CS : 101 myths debunked / Brenda R. Affinati.
    p. ; cm.
  New USMLE step 2 clinical skills
  ISBN 978-0-07-182813-0 (pbk.)—ISBN 0-07-182813-3 (pbk.)
  I. Title. II. Title: New USMLE step 2 clinical skills.
  [DNLM: 1. Physical Examination—methods—Problems and Exercises.
2. Clinical Competence—Problems and Exercises. WB 18.2]
  RB38.25
  616.07'5076—dc23
                                                                        2013039327

International Edition ISBN 978-1-25-925142-9; MHID 1-25-925142-X.
Copyright © 2014. Exclusive rights by McGraw-Hill Education, for manufacture and export. This book cannot be re-exported from the country to which it is consigned by McGraw-Hill Education. The International Edition is not available in North America.

McGraw-Hill Education books are available at special quantity discounts to use as premiums and sales promotions, or for use in corporate training programs. To contact a representative please visit the Contact Us pages at www.mhprofessional.com.

Dedication

To my mom, who always encouraged
and supported my dreams.

To my wonderful husband, Mario, and our three
amazing boys; Jordan, Joshua and Justin.
Thank you for your love and support.

Contents

Introduction

Welcome to "Debunking the Myths." Let's make your preparation for the new USMLE Step 2 CS Exam fun. How? By getting straightforward answers to your most common questions and concerns. The Step 2 CS exam is unlike any other USMLE exam. It is NOT a simple multiple-choice test. You cannot simply memorize medical facts to pass this exam. The Step 2 CS exam is an interactive test that involves standardized patients. Most students feel uncomfortable dealing with "fake" patients; however, the method of standardized patient-based testing has been validated internationally.

Why am I calling it "New"? Recently the Step 2 CS exam changed in two significant ways.

1. In 2012, a new section was added to the patient note. In this new section, the examinee must list the positive and negative findings from the history and physical examination. This has led to general confusion about how to support a diagnosis. Prior to the change, formulating a differential diagnosis was enough. With the addition of listing supportive data for each diagnosis, the USMLE is challenging you to defend your diagnosis with the proof you obtained during the encounter. This is a wonderful way to reinforce the diagnostic thought process every young physician must learn.

2. In 2013, the USMLE changed the minimum passing requirement for two of the three Step 2 CS subcomponents: Communication and Interpersonal Skills (CIS) and Integrated Clinical Encounter (ICE). This change will significantly lower the overall pass rate. The USMLE has estimated that the overall pass rate could drop as much as 18% for international medical graduates and as much as 3% for US medical students.

The importance of passing all the USMLE exams on the first attempt is critical; a failure will significantly affect your ability to secure a residency position in the United States. However, I still encounter students and graduates who neglect their preparation for the Step 2 CS. They are convinced it is a simple straightforward pass/fail exam. I believe that it is, but you need to be aware of how your performance is being evaluated. The idea to write this book came from you. Over my years of teaching US medical students and international medical graduates, I have jotted down the common questions and concerns. In this book, I am sharing with you the recurrent misconceptions about the Step 2 CS exam. My goal is to debunk these myths. Once your mind is clear of these myths, you will be free to prepare for this exam both efficiently and productively, and ultimately pass!

The book is divided into four sections. The first three sections are the separate subcomponents of the CS exam: Communication and Interpersonal Skills (CIS), Integrated Clinical Encounter (ICE), and Spoken English Proficiency (SEP). You must pass each of these three subcomponents in order to pass this exam. If you fail one subcomponent, you fail the entire exam. Essentially, you are taking three tests in one day. The fourth section deals with miscellaneous myths.

CIS Myths

Fostering the Relationship

Myth # 1
"I don't have time to knock before entering the room."

Debunking the myth:
Knocking is courteous, and you should always knock prior to entering the room. Simply knock and enter. The only exceptions are the telephone cases. There are no standardized patients in the room for the telephone cases; therefore, there is no need to knock.

Myth # 2
"Introducing myself is not important. Besides, I don't have enough time for it!"

Debunking the myth:

Upon entering the room, you must take the time to introduce yourself. Greet the patient by name and introduce yourself, giving your name. Use a formal title to address the patient. Avoid using first names except with children or adolescents. For example, "Hello Mr. Jones?" (pause for reply) "I'm Dr. Smith and I'll be the doctor taking care of you today."

The introduction is an essential step in fostering the relationship with the patient. You must know the patient's preferred name and the patient must know your name. It is critical that you begin the encounter with the introduction. The introduction is the foundation of the doctor–patient relationship. You may introduce yourself however you wish, as either a medical student or as a doctor. You may introduce yourself using your real name. And, please do not mention the name of your school or institution.

Myth # 3
"I don't really need to know the patient's name."

Debunking the myth:
Yes you do! Write the patient's name at the top of your blank sheet of paper prior to entering the room. While you are performing the history and physical, you will be jotting down notes. Each time you do, you'll see the patient's name.

Throughout the encounter, feel free to use his/her name. By doing this, you'll be strengthening the doctor–patient relationship and promoting an atmosphere of trust.

Myth # 4
"I need to shake the patient's hand to get an extra point."

Debunking the myth:
It is not necessary to shake the patient's hand during the introduction. You will not receive "extra points" for hand shaking.

Myth # 5
"Establishing eye contact is not important, besides it makes me feel uncomfortable."

Debunking the myth:
Establishing eye contact with your patient is critical in developing the doctor–patient relationship. Patients feel their doctor is uninterested if eye contact is not established and maintained throughout the encounter. The standardized patients are trained intensively to observe your nonverbal cues, such as establishing eye contact. If eye contact is not established, the patient feels the doctor may be uninterested in their care.

Myth # 6
"I don't really need to listen to the patient."

Debunking the myth:

You need to actively listen to each of the patients. Active listening requires you to pay close attention to what the patient is saying, being alert to the patient's emotional state, and using verbal and nonverbal skills to motivate the patient to elaborate on their story. Active listening creates a secure environment for the patient to share personal information. So stop worrying about how much time you have left in the 15-minute encounter and focus your concentration on listening to the patient.

Myth # 7
"I don't really need to bond with the patients."

Debunking the myth:
One of the most valued skills in clinical medicine is the ability to relate effectively with patients. In order to obtain the patient's story, you need to use techniques that promote trust and convey respect. This supportive interaction helps place the patient at ease when sharing their information and it is the foundation of the doctor–patient relationship.

Myth # 8
"I don't see how my posture can affect my score on the Step 2 CS exam."

Debunking the myth:
Studies have found that the posture of the doctor is influential in determining how much information the patient shares during a typical encounter. If you are sitting, you should lean forward, and do not fold your arms across your chest. It's also useful to nod your head to encourage the patient to talk.

Whether it's conscious or not, you send messages through your words AND your behavior. Posture, eye contact, gestures, and tone of voice all reveal your true intentions and interests.

Myth # 9
"I heard it's ok to wear scrubs to the Step 2 CS exam."

Debunking the myth:
You need to wear comfortable, yet professional, clothing. Hospital scrubs should only be worn in the hospital. Professional clothing can be considered dress pants (no jeans), dress shirts (no T-shirts), and dress shoes (no tennis shoes).

Myth # 10
"My hands literally shake when I'm nervous. I'm sure I'll lose a point for it."

Debunking the myth:
Everyone experiences nervous energy. Rest assured, you will neither be the first nor the last examinee to experience shaky hands. Standardized patients are aware this happens. It is a very common reaction. Try not to focus on it. Ignore your trembling hands and focus on the patient.

Myth # 11

"No one should tolerate a drug abuser or alcoholic. They need criticizing from their doctor, or else they will never change."

Debunking the myth:

You should never criticize your patient, even if you feel the behavior is dreadful and shocking. You need to be consistently respectful and nonjudgmental during every patient encounter.

Myth # 12
"If the patient goes off on a tangent, I need to interrupt her to redirect the interview."

Debunking the myth:
I doubt you will ever need to interrupt a patient on the Step 2 Clinical Skills (CS) exam. The standardized patients rarely elaborate unnecessarily. If you feel they are babbling, I would encourage you to listen (and not interrupt). The answer to the case is most likely hidden in that babble!

Myth # 13
"There should never be a silent moment during the interview."

Debunking the myth:
It is perfectly appropriate to have silent pauses during a medical interview. It frequently occurs when the physician takes a moment to process the information that has been obtained. If you feel uncomfortable doing this, then simply tell the patient, "Let me take a moment to sort through everything you've told me. I want to make sure that I'm not missing anything." Patients prefer to have a thoughtful and thorough physician over a hasty and superficial one.

Myth # 14

"I think the drape is just a big waste of time. I don't know why they have it in the room."

Debunking the myth:

The drape is like a blanket. It is used to protect the patient's dignity. Keep the patient covered (draped) until you are ready to examine a particular area. Once you've finished, then remember to re-cover the patient.

Myth # 15
"I have to smile, no matter what."

Debunking the myth:
You do not need to smile, so don't worry about forcing it (or worse yet, faking it). However, you must be polite, approachable, and respectful. If the standardized patient is good humored and friendly, you will smile naturally.

2

Gathering Information

Myth # 16
"The patient must sit down before I can take a history."

Debunking the myth:
In order for you to obtain a complete history, the patient needs to feel at ease. In some instances, the patient may be nervous, angry, or upset and may insist on standing or pacing around the room. It's reasonable for you to ask the patient if they'd be more comfortable sitting during the interview. However, if the patient refuses, it's okay. Go ahead and take the history while the patient is standing or pacing. As the interview progresses and you create a relationship with the patient, they may eventually sit down.

Myth # 17
"The presenting complaint is usually unrelated to the final diagnosis."

Debunking the myth:

The presenting complaint is critical in helping you develop the final diagnosis. The exam is designed to evaluate your ability to collect information that is important for a patient's presenting complaint. When you are analyzing the examinee instructions prior to entering the room, you need to develop a differential diagnosis, taking into account the chief complaint, age, gender, and vital signs. I recommend that you write this differential on your blank sheet of paper while you're still outside the room.

Once you enter the room, introduce yourself. Then start the medical history by asking the patient an open-ended question related to the presenting complaint. Listen carefully and take notes as needed. Refer to your list of preliminary diagnoses and start generating pertinent questions to help you rule in and rule out each one. These pertinent questions will ultimately help you discover the final diagnosis. And remember, each pertinent question you ask is a "point" on the Communication and Interpersonal Skills (CIS) Gathering Information portion of the exam.

Myth # 18
"All the patients are presenting with an acute problem."

Debunking the myth:
There is a mix of acute and chronic cases on the exam. Be prepared to handle either situation.

Myth # 19
"I don't have time on this exam to ask open-ended questions."

Debunking the myth:

After introducing yourself, I highly recommend that you start the medical interview with an open-ended question. For example, "I know you are here for shoulder pain, can you tell me more about it?" As the interview progresses, you should shift to the more specific questions (or closed-ended questions) to help narrow your diagnosis. Here are two examples of a closed-ended question:

- "Can you tell me when it started?"
- "Can you show me exactly where it hurts?"

Myth # 20
"Trying to figure out the chronological order of events when obtaining the history will take too much time."

Debunking the myth:
You need to obtain a history of present illness (HPI) on each case. The HPI is the complete and chronological account of the presenting complaint. Without knowing the chronology of the complaints, you will have a difficult time narrowing down the diagnosis. If the presenting complaint is pain, you need to find out when the pain started, whether it is getting better or worse, if the pain comes and goes, etc. By the time you finish taking the history, you should be able to draw a timeline of the presenting complaint.

Myth # 21

"It's ok to ask the patient: "You're not having any chest pain, are you?"

Debunking the myth:

No, it's not OK. Asking a question that suggests your desired response is a leading question. The above question is a perfect example of a leading question. You must *avoid* using leading questions on the Step 2 CS exam. Instead, ask: "Are you having any chest pain?"

Myth # 22
"Paraphrasing is a big waste of time."

Debunking the myth:
In the context of taking a patient's medical history, paraphrasing is when you reword your patient's answers using different words to provide greater clarity. Paraphrasing demonstrates that you *listened* to your patient and that you *understood* what they said. Listening to and understanding your patient are the key components of the doctor–patient relationship. The patient needs to know that you are listening and understanding in order for them to trust you. And if by chance you misunderstood what was said, paraphrasing provides the patient an opportunity to correct you.

Myth # 23
"I can ask a series of questions very quickly and get a bunch of extra points."

Debunking the myth:
You must not ask more than one question at a time. Asking a series of questions is generally confusing for the patient. Here is an example: "Any nausea, vomiting, diarrhea, weight loss, or blood in your stool?"

Asking more than one question at a time may lead to a negative answer, which may or may not be true. If the above five questions are important to ask for your case, then you'll need to ask each one separately, "Do you have any of the following complaints, Nausea?" (pause) "Vomiting?" (pause) "Diarrhea?" (pause) etc.

Myth # 24

"I definitely should NOT encourage the patient to talk. This will waste way too much time!"

Debunking the myth:

You need to encourage the patient to explain the situation in their own words. Using phrases like, "Tell me more about it…" invites the patient to tell their story. Continue to encourage the patient to talk. Feel free to use phrases like "Go on," or "Mm-hmm." This will encourage the patient to give you more information. Do not interrupt the patient and do not inject any new information. Simply listen and acknowledge their story.

Myth # 25
"I have to counsel every patient who drinks alcohol."

Debunking the myth:
It is socially acceptable in the United States for healthy adults to drink alcohol (men 2 drinks/day, women 1 drink/day). (A "drink" equals one 12 oz beer or one 5 oz glass of wine or 1.5 oz of liquor.) Counseling is not necessary in these adults. However, alcohol use is contraindicated in many medical situations. Some examples are pregnancy, jaundice, history of liver disease, and cirrhosis. If your patient has a medical situation for which alcohol is contraindicated, then you need to counsel the patient on cessation/abstinence.

Myth # 26
"I have to ask the CAGE questions on every patient who drinks any amount of alcohol."

Debunking the myth:
It is socially acceptable for a man to have 2 "drinks" a day or an average of 14/week and a woman to have 1 "drink" a day or an average of 7/week. You do not have to ask the CAGE questions in these patients.

A "drink" is defined as

- 1 shot of hard liquor = 1.5 ounces
- 1 glass of wine = 5 ounces
- 1 glass/can of beer = 12 ounces

If your patient drinks more than the socially acceptable limits, then you should ask the CAGE questions to screen for alcohol abuse. The CAGE questions are as follows:

1. Have you ever felt the need to **C**ut down on drinking?
2. Have you ever felt **A**nnoyed by criticism of your drinking?
3. Have you ever felt **G**uilty about drinking?
4. Have you ever taken a drink first thing in the morning (**E**ye-opener) to steady your nerves or get over a hangover?

If your patient answers affirmatively to two or more of the questions, you should suspect alcohol abuse or dependence. You should counsel the patient on the adverse effects of alcohol misuse.

Myth # 27
"Asking the CAGE questions on all of my patients will give me extra points."

Debunking the myth:
If you ask the CAGE questions on healthy patients who are drinking socially acceptable amounts of alcohol, you are simply wasting your time. You will not receive extra points for asking unnecessary questions.

Myth # 28
"I have to ask every patient their family history."

Debunking the myth:
The cases on the Step 2 CS exam are focused encounters. The patient is presenting with a chief complaint or concern. Obtaining a family history is not necessary on each encounter. Family history should be asked when you suspect a disease that may have a familial predisposition. Common examples are cancer, heart disease, diabetes, hypertension, hypothyroidism, depression, asthma, and migraines. If a woman presents with depression, weight gain, irregular periods, dry skin, and hair loss, you would definitely want to ask about a family history of thyroid problems.

Myth # 29
"I have to ask every patient their surgical history (or their sexual history)."

Debunking the myth:
Remember, each of the CS encounters is focused. You should only ask a surgical or sexual history if it is pertinent for your case.

Myth # 30
"All patients need to be asked about tobacco use."

Debunking the myth:
While it's true that tobacco increases the risk for a number of health issues, the cases on the Step 2 CS exam are focused encounters. You should ask about tobacco use if it's pertinent for your case. If your patient is complaining of a cough, clearly knowing about tobacco use would be important information in developing the differential diagnosis.

3

Providing Information

Myth # 31
"I don't have time to summarize the information for the patient at the end of the encounter."

Debunking the myth:
You must provide a summary at the end of each encounter.
Summarizing the information is a critical part of your CIS score. Your summary should include the following:

1. A brief synopsis of the history you obtained

2. Pertinent physical exam findings

3. A brief differential diagnosis in layman's terms

4. Diagnostic tests you plan to order (again, in layman's terms!)

5. Ask if they have any questions

6. If they have a question, be sure to answer it!

Myth # 32
"I was told in a review course that I need to mention three diagnoses during the summary."

Debunking the myth:
There is no need to force yourself to mention three (or more) differentials. What you need to do is give an explanation of the diagnoses you are considering (using layman's terms) and what studies you plan to order.

Myth # 33
"Most patients understand words like frequency, dysuria, and nocturia."

Debunking the myth:

Most patients speak and read at the level of a teenager. The above terms are examples of medical jargon and they are unfamiliar to the general population. When physicians use medical jargon, they jeopardize their ability to communicate with the patient. If the patient does not understand the obscure language, they will not be able to make educated decisions with regard to their medical care.

Here's an example of an *unacceptable* summary:

"Mrs. Peters, it sounds like you had a *syncopal* event. It may have been caused by an *arrhythmia*. I'll need to order an *ECG* and *2D ECHO STAT*."

Although you may have come up with the correct diagnosis and workup in the case (Integrated Clinical Encounter score), you undermined your ability to communicate with the patient (CIS score). Poor Mrs. Peters has no idea what's wrong with her and what you plan to do about it.

Let's try it again, this time avoiding the unusual terms:

"Mrs. Peters, it sounds like you passed out. This may have been caused by a problem with your heart. I'll need to order a test that checks the rhythm of your heart and another test to take a good look at how your heart is working. I plan on getting these tests done right away. Do you have any questions?"

Myth # 34
"I should not encourage the patient to ask me questions."

Debunking the myth:
You need to encourage your patient to ask questions! The patients are grading your ability to encourage and answer questions. Even if you are led to believe that the patient understands (by nodding his/her head), it's still important to ask if they have any questions. There are many reasons why they are reluctant to ask questions: embarrassment, fear, confusion, and feeling overwhelmed. Regardless of the reason, if you open the door for questions, the patient will undoubtedly feel at ease to ask.

4

Helping the Patient Make Decisions

Myth # 35
"I do not have to discuss my diagnostic workup with the patient. Besides, I won't have enough time."

Debunking the myth:
After discussing the diagnostic possibilities, you need to review the diagnostic studies you plan to order (using layman's terms). Then, inquire if the patient has any questions. If the patient expresses a concern, you need to address it as you would in a normal clinical setting.

Myth # 36
"I've heard there are some cases on the exam that are just too complicated. On these cases, I should postpone making any medical decisions or ordering a diagnostic workup."

Debunking the myth:
It is possible that you'll encounter a case that seems too complicated for your level of training. Although these cases were created for medical students in their final years, you may feel bewildered by a patient's complaints. If this occurs, you should not defer any decision making to others. You need to imagine yourself as the only provider available, and you need to do the best you can to figure it out.

If, after the history and physical, you are clueless (the diagnosis eludes you), I'm going to offer you some practical advice that will ultimately help raise your score. First, take a minute to reflect. This is easily done by telling the patient you need a moment to review your notes to be sure you haven't forgotten anything. During this time, scrutinize the information you've already obtained during the history. (Your notes on the blank sheet of paper are critical for this step.) Take a deep breath and open your mind to other diagnostic possibilities. I'm sure at this point, you'll discover a few important questions that you neglected to ask. The answer to one of these questions may be the key to solving the case. Even if you can't solve the case, you'll probably gain a few extra points for your CIS score under Data Gathering.

Myth # 37

"If the patient refuses to accept my plan of action for their care, they are just trying to distract me to make me fail the exam."

Debunking the myth:

The patients on the Step 2 CS exam cannot choose to fail you. They are simply playing a role. The cases are written to test your ability to manage difficult situations. Toward the end of the encounter, when you are discussing the diagnostic workup, the patient may refuse the tests you are recommending. If the patient rejects your plan of action, it's your duty to figure out why. Gently and compassionately ask the patient about their concerns. Possible reasons could be their social, emotional, or economic situation. You'll need to be prepared to respond appropriately. Here are some examples:

- Lack of information: "I don't understand why you want to order this test." *Patiently explain why the test is needed.*

- Emotional difficulties: "I'm scared it will show that I have cancer." *Explain that whatever the test reveals, you'll be with them every step of the way.*

- Insufficient financial resources: "I lost my job last month, and I don't have medical insurance to pay for any of this." *Your office staff will develop a reasonable financial plan.*

The influence of these issues is significantly reduced through effective communication between you and the patient. Once you understand the patient's anxieties and concerns, you can start formulating a mutual plan of action ... and go on to pass the exam!

5

Supporting Emotions

Myth # 38

"My job is to figure out the final diagnosis. It's not important to discuss how the illness impacts the patient's life. Especially since these are all "fake patients" anyway!"

Debunking the myth:

Ultimately, you want to figure out the most likely diagnosis, but you also have to be sensitive to the patient's emotional state. If the patient appears to be in distress, that is, anxious or depressed, it is your job to acknowledge the emotional clues. Patients tend to withhold their concerns verbally, but they give you nonverbal clues. By acknowledging and responding to these clues, you'll build a stronger rapport with the patient and ultimately understand the impact the illness has on the patient's life. Respond immediately when you hear or sense an emotional clue. For example, in response to an emotional clue from a patient you may respond, "It's understandable that you'd feel that way," or "This must be very difficult for you."

Myth # 39
"It's impossible to feel empathy when I know the patient is faking their symptoms."

Debunking the myth:
Empathy has always been considered an essential component of compassionate care. The whole point of empathy is to focus your attention on the patient and acknowledge their emotions. Empathy facilitates the doctor–patient relationship and builds trust. The trust enables the patient to feel more comfortable and give a fuller history.

On the Step 2 CS exam, the patients are only portraying a medical illness. Therefore, it may be difficult for you to "portray empathy" in return. Regardless of this fact, you need to move beyond it. Try to imagine that all of the patients are real. This will be easier than you think. The standardized patients are well-trained actors. During the exam, you'll feel like it's an actual patient encounter. Accept this feeling and respond to each of the patients as you normally would. If your thoughts start drifting ("Everything this patient says is fake. I'm sure I'm going to fail. I'm running out of time. Oh my gosh, why am I here?"), you stop focusing your attention on the patient. Stop the inner mental dialogue immediately and start listening to the patient.

Myth # 40
"Inquiring about the support system is a waste of time."

Debunking the myth:

Our support system is the network of family and friends that provide us with emotional, social, and economic support. We all tap into our support system when we are in the midst of a difficult situation. A strong support system helps us cope. If you encounter a patient on the Step 2 CS exam going through a difficult time, inquiring about their support system could be beneficial. The fact that you discovered it and helped the patient find a solution could possibly avert a disaster. (And, of course, increase your chances of passing!)

Myth # 41
"If a patient yells at me, I know I'm going to fail the exam."

Debunking the myth:

If a patient yells at you, it is most likely "part of the script" for the case. In other words, the USMLE knows that these situations can occur in real life, and they are testing your ability to manage very difficult situations. Anger is a difficult emotion to handle, in any situation. My suggestion for you is to stay calm (never get angry or yell at a patient). Try to figure out why the patient is so angry, and once you understand the source of the anger, you'll be better equipped to deal with the situation.

ICE Myths

6

Developing the Differential Diagnosis

Myth # 42
"I don't have time to read the Examinee Instructions on the doorway prior to entering the room."

Debunking the myth:

You *must* take the time to read the Examinee Instructions prior to entering the room. The USMLE is providing you with vital information to help you tackle the case logically. If you take the time to analyze this information (age, gender, chief complaint, and vitals), you'll be prepared to ask pertinent questions during the history.

Once you hear the announcement that the encounter has begun, I suggest that you spend at least 1 or 2 minutes reading the Examinee Instructions. Jot down the patient's name, the chief complaint, and the vitals on the blank sheet of paper. Start formulating and listing diagnoses at this time.

Myth # 43
"The blank sheet of paper is not very useful."

Debunking the myth:
The blank sheet of paper is extremely useful, if you use it wisely. Once you hear the announcement that the patient encounter has begun, start reading/analyzing the Examinee Instructions. Take your time. Write down the patient's name at the top of the paper. (You know that you'll forget it once you walk into the room.) Under the patient's name, list the gender (M or F), age, and vitals (or at the very least, the abnormal vitals). When it is time for you to type your patient note, this information will be readily available for you to transcribe.

As I stated in myth no. 42, start listing your preliminary diagnoses. When you organize your thoughts using the blank sheet of paper in this manner, you'll be prepared to ask the focused questions required to ultimately discover the final diagnosis.

Once you are in the room taking the patient's history, continue taking notes. We all tend to forget information we obtain when we are under stressful conditions (like taking the Step 2 CS exam!). Referring to your notes will also help prevent you from repeating a question you already asked.

The blank sheet of paper is a gift from the USMLE! You need to take advantage of it.

One last word on the blank sheet of paper: it is collected at the end of each encounter, but it is not scored.

Myth # 44
"I won't be able to figure out the diagnosis from the history."

Debunking the myth:

This is absolutely a myth! Every practicing physician agrees that the most important aspect of a patient encounter is the history. In most cases, the medical history provides enough information to make an initial diagnosis. The physicians and medical educators who develop the cases for the Step 2 CS exam know this. The exam is written to assess your ability to pursue possible diagnoses during the medical history. Being able to take a focused medical history is essential for passing this exam.

Myth # 45
"The patients complaining of fatigue are hypothyroid, anemic, or depressed."

Debunking the myth:
When I teach students and residents about fatigue, I ask them to give me the differential. Every single time, they list the same three diagnoses: hypothyroidism, anemia, and depression. And then, they stop. This is a common error. Unfortunately, it may lead you to eliminate or never consider other equally likely diagnoses. When working through a case of fatigue, it's best to keep your mind wide open to any possibility. As you ask pertinent questions (depending on the age, gender, and vitals), you'll start unraveling the diagnosis. If your mind is set on making the diagnosis of hypothyroidism, anemia, or depression, you won't recognize the actual diagnosis.

Don't make a square peg fit in a circle hole. If the symptoms don't fit the diagnosis, then you probably have the wrong diagnosis. Take a mental step back, rethink the case, open your mind, and ask more questions!

One last point on fatigue: over 90% of the time, you'll obtain the diagnosis from the medical history alone. So expect to spend more time taking the history than on the physical exam.

Myth # 46
"I'm worried about the zebras."

Debunking the myth:
Zebras don't live in the United States, horses do! If your patient is complaining of loss of sensation in the hands and feet, think of a horse (diabetes), not a zebra (beriberi).

7

Performing the Physical Exam

Myth # 47
"I can pretend to wash my hands before I perform the physical exam."

Debunking the myth:
Do not ever pretend to wash your hands. You need to observe proper hygiene with the patients during the Step 2 CS exam, as you would in the care of real patients.

Myth # 48
"I'll need to recheck the vital signs in each case."

Debunking the myth:
The USMLE clearly states that it is not necessary to repeat them, unless you believe it is specifically required. However, keep in mind that you should *only* consider the vital signs that were originally listed on the Examinee Instructions when developing your diagnoses and diagnostic workup.

Let's be realistic here. The USMLE is not going to be able to make a standardized patient become orthostatic. Even if the patient is complaining of vomiting and diarrhea for the past week, they clearly don't "really" have these symptoms, otherwise they would not have been able to come to work as a standardized patient! The standardized patients are actors and they are generally in good health. They are simply portraying an illness. So if you spend the time checking orthostatic in a patient with vomiting and diarrhea, I can guarantee they won't be orthostatic. Your job on the exam is to figure out the diagnosis, not worry about treatment (like how much normal saline the patient will need to restore their fluid volume)!

Myth # 49

"I should develop my differential diagnosis around the patient's actual vital signs, not the vital signs from the Examinee Instructions."

Debunking the myth:

The USMLE has carefully and logically constructed each case in the exam. The Examinee Instructions are part of that structure and are within the control of the USMLE. The standardized patients are highly trained individuals; however, they are not expected to simulate the vital signs listed in the Examinee Instructions. This would be impossible. *You should only use the vital signs from the Examinee Instructions in formulating your differential diagnosis.*

Bottom line: Do *not* recheck the vitals, unless you are specifically instructed to do so in the Examinee Instructions.

Myth # 50
"I can "fake" the physical exam maneuvers. I'll still get the points even if I just go through the motions."

Debunking the myth:
Do not fake the physical exam maneuvers. In fact, you need to perform the maneuvers correctly in order to get credit. The standardized patients are extensively trained to know the proper maneuvers. If you try to cut corners on the physical exam in order to save time, you are making a critical error. If the maneuver was pertinent for that case, you will only get the point if you perform the maneuver as you would in a real clinical encounter.

Myth # 51
"I need to examine as many organ systems as possible to get enough points to pass."

Debunking the myth:

More is not always better! You need to be focused! Each case is developed to elicit a process of history taking and physical examination maneuvers in order to assess your ability to pursue several reasonable diagnoses. If you spend your time examining areas that are not pertinent for the case, you are not getting extra points. You are simply wasting your time.

Myth # 52
"If the patient clearly has a pneumonia, I should document in the patient note that I heard rales on the lung exam."

Debunking the myth:
Do not write in your patient note what you *expect* to find on the physical exam. Only document your *actual* findings. For example, if the patient has the classic presentation for a pneumonia, you'd expect to have positive findings on the lung exam (like rales/crackles). If you listen to the lungs properly and they are clear, then you should document that in your patient note. (Lungs—clear to auscultation bilaterally.)

Although you'd expect to have positive findings on the physical exam, you should only document the findings that are actually present. Do not make up findings.

On the flip side, you need to realize that the patients are going to be simulating physical exam findings! For example, the patient may mimic rales/crackles while you are listening to their lungs. If this occurs, you need to accept the finding as real and document it in the physical exam portion of your note. You should also use that as a positive physical exam finding to support your diagnosis of pneumonia.

Myth # 53

"If my patient had a stroke, I'll need to do a full neurological exam."

Debunking the myth:

You will never have time to do a complete neurological exam on the Step 2 CS exam. Your focused physical exam will be based on the patient's presenting complaint and the information you obtained during the history.

Myth # 54

"If the patient's presenting complaint is bloody stools, I will "go through the motions" of a rectal exam, but I won't really do it."

Debunking the myth:

You will never "go through the motions" on any portion of this exam. And you will *never* perform a rectal exam on a standardized patient. If you feel it is indicated, you can discuss the plan with the patient and list the rectal exam in diagnostic studies at the end of the patient note.

Myth # 55

"On certain cases, I will need to perform a breast exam."

Debunking the myth:

You will *never* perform a rectal, pelvic, inguinal hernia, genitourinary, female breast, corneal reflex exam, or throat swab during the Step 2 CS exam. If any one of these exams is indicated, list it in your diagnostic studies.

Myth # 56
"During the physical exam, it's ok to push harder if necessary."

Debunking the myth:
You should *never* use unnecessary force while examining the patients. You will obtain the information you need by applying the appropriate pressure during the maneuvers.

Be especially attentive during the otoscopic exam and using the tongue depressor to examine the throat.

Myth # 57
"I can't perform a physical exam on an adolescent without the parent's consent."

Debunking the myth:

Except for the restricted maneuvers, you automatically have consent to perform a physical exam on every patient, even adolescents.

Myth # 58
"I can't ask any history questions during the physical exam."

Debunking the myth:
YES you can! While you're examining the patient, you may think of additional history questions that you neglected to ask. Feel free to ask these questions while you are performing the physical exam.

8

Writing the Patient Note

Myth # 59
"If I finish the encounter early and leave the room, I can always go back in if I forgot something."

Debunking the myth:

If you leave the encounter early, you will have extra time to type your note. You will not, however, be allowed to return inside the room for any reason. If you re-enter, it will be considered misconduct.

If you finish the encounter early, I suggest that you ask yourself one question before leaving—"Do I know the most likely diagnosis?" If you can't answer with a strong YES, then check your notes and start asking the patient more pertinent questions. Be satisfied that you obtained all the necessary information before you leave the room.

Myth # 60
"I'm not very good at typing, but this exam is testing my medical knowledge, not how fast I type."

Debunking the myth:
If your typing skills are poor, I strongly suggest taking a typing course. Typing confidently will decrease your anxiety during the exam. You will have 10 minutes to type the note, and if you type slowly, you may run out of time.

Myth # 61
"The layout of the keyboard is not important."

Debunking the myth:
Prior to the exam, you need to practice typing your patient notes using a US keyboard layout. If you regularly use a different layout prior to the exam, you will make errors while typing your patient note. This will cause needless anxiety and will inhibit your ability to process the case and develop an appropriate differential diagnosis.

Myth # 62
"Since I already frequently type patient notes, I do not need to practice typing notes prior to the exam."

Debunking the myth:
Although you may already feel comfortable typing patient notes, I guarantee that you are not comfortable using the USMLE format. The USMLE has provided a simulation of the program used for writing patient notes. It is located at http://www.usmle.org/practice-materials/step-2-cs/patient-note-practice2.html. I recommend that you practice typing mock patient notes everyday on the website prior to taking the exam.

Myth # 63

"I can use any abbreviation in the patient note."

Debunking the myth:

The use of abbreviations is invaluable. Abbreviations assist you in documenting the pertinent data in an effective and efficient manner. However, the improper use of abbreviations could adversely affect your score. I have frequently witnessed the inaccurate use of abbreviations, especially with international medical graduates. The USMLE provides a list of commonly used abbreviations in its *Step 2 Clinical Skills (CS) Content Description and General Information* brochure (available online at usmle.org.). Please study this list, and realize although it is not a *complete* list, it illustrates the common abbreviations used in the United States.

Myth # 64
"My handwriting is atrocious. I'm thrilled to type all the patient notes."

Debunking the myth:
It is possible for the examination center to experience technical difficulties with the patient note software. If this occurs, typing the patient note will not be an option. You will be required to write the patient note by hand. You need to be prepared for this possibility. If your writing is illegible, it will adversely impact your score. Write as neatly as possible.

Myth # 65

"If I run out of space while typing my history, I can finish it in the physical exam section."

Debunking the myth:

Do not put any history in the physical exam section of the note. You will not receive credit for that portion of the history. There are two reasons this can occur.

1. *You have too much useless information in your history.* This routinely occurs because examinees are convinced that "more is better." The "more is better" philosophy is wrong. You only need to list the information that is pertinent to the case.

2. *You ran out of lines.* How could that possibly happen? Well, you have 950 characters, but only 15 lines! If you hit the return button after each symptom, it will look like this:

   headache
   fever
   numbness
   tingling
   weakness

You just used 5 out of your 15 lines limit, even though it's only 37 characters.

Instead, you should list them horizontally (without hitting the return button), like this:

   headache, fever, numbness, tingling, weakness

(40 characters and only 1 line.)

Myth # 66

"Since I only have 10 minutes, I should type all the information I obtained as fast as possible and not worry about the overall structure of the patient note."

Debunking the myth:

Trained physicians rate your patient note. Your score is not only based on documenting the pertinent positive and negative findings from the encounter but also the quality of documentation. The patient note is a scientific and legal document, so it needs to be clear and intelligible. Patient notes have a specific structure. Subjective data (what the patient tells you) belong to the history section. Objective data (what you detect during the physical exam) belong to the physical exam section. It's essential that you write patient notes that are clear and easy to follow.

Myth # 67
"How I write the history doesn't really matter, as long as I've included all the important information."

Debunking the myth:
You are scored on your ability to organize the history you obtained. The subjective data is organized in a typical way. The first line should include the patient's name, age, gender, and chief complaint. The next few lines should be the history of present illness in chronological order, including pertinent positives and negatives from the review of systems. Finally, you'll list pertinent past medical history, past surgical history, meds, family history, and social history. Labeling each of these sections increases the clarity of your note.

The physical exam (objective data) also needs to flow. First, list the vitals and a general description of the patient. Next, list the pertinent physical exam findings you performed during the encounter starting with the head and going down to the toes (ie, HEENT, Pulm, CV, Abd, Ext, and Neuro).

Be careful not to let subjective items stray into the physical exam section, or vice versa.

Myth # 68
"I should never leave the physical exam section of the note blank."

Debunking the myth:
It's impossible to perform a physical exam during the telephone encounters; so in these types of cases, leave the physical exam section of the note blank.

Myth # 69

"I can put physical exam maneuvers in my patient note, even if I didn't perform them during the encounter."

Debunking the myth:

When you are typing the physical examination portion of your note, you should only include the parts of the physical examination that you performed during the encounter. Do not include maneuvers that you did not perform in the room. Do not list maneuvers that you would have performed if you had more time.

Myth # 70

"If they say to stop typing, it's ok for me to finish my sentence first."

Debunking the myth:

Immediately hit "Submit" when you hear the announcement to stop typing. If you continue to type, it will be considered misconduct.

9

Data Interpretation

Myth # 71
"I need to list the most fatal diagnosis first."

Debunking the myth:
Although it's tempting to list the deadliest disease first, the USMLE clearly instructs you to list the *most likely* diagnosis first. Use the information you obtained from the history and physical and list the diagnosis with the highest probability of being the true cause of the patient's complaint first. List your remaining diagnoses in order of likelihood. If a diagnosis is not likely (even if it's fatal), you should not list it.

Myth # 72
"I will always need to list three diagnoses in the data interpretation section of the patient note."

Debunking the myth:
Only list the diagnoses that remain possible after performing a pertinent history and physical exam. Do not force yourself to add ridiculous diagnoses. It will only make you look ridiculous!

Myth # 73
"If I list myocardial infarction on my differential diagnosis on each case of "chest pain" I'll get extra points."

Debunking the myth:

The differential diagnosis of chest pain is extensive, and it does include myocardial infarction. However, after you've taken the history and performed the physical exam, a myocardial infarction may not be likely. Here's an example: your patient is a young healthy female. She complains of a cough, fever, and chest pain. When you take her history, you discover that her cough and fever preceded the chest pain, and she only has the chest pain when she coughs. On exam, the chest pain is reproducible. You would list costochondritis as your first diagnosis. You wouldn't list myocardial infarction at all!

10

Supporting the Diagnosis

Myth # 74
"It's impossible to support each of my diagnoses."

Debunking the myth:
If you've performed a pertinent history and physical, and you can't support the diagnosis, then you should not list the diagnosis.

In 2012, the USMLE added a "Supporting the diagnosis" section because examinees tended to list diagnoses that were improbable for a particular case. Very popular Step 2 CS review courses actually taught the mantra: "List five to stay alive!" (At that time, it was possible to list up to five diagnoses.) I was thrilled when the USMLE modified the exam to require examinees to support their diagnosis with information obtained from the history and physical exam. It's a simple attempt to prevent you from listing diagnoses that are far-fetched and unrealistic. In other words, if there is no information to support the diagnosis, then the diagnosis is not likely and should not be listed.

Myth # 75
"Since I really don't understand "Supporting the diagnosis" section, I'm just going to skip it."

Debunking the myth:
Do not skip any section of the patient note. I'll try to explain this section in simple terms so you can increase your Integrated Clinical Encounter (ICE) score.

Most illnesses have common presenting symptoms. When you group the symptoms, you are able to recognize the diagnosis. While preparing for this exam, study the common presenting symptoms for common and important diseases that occur in the United States.

The presence of symptoms (positive findings) helps support a diagnosis. The absence of symptoms (negative findings) can also help support a diagnosis.

Myth # 76
"Negative Findings can't help support the diagnosis."

Debunking the myth:
The absence of a symptom (negative finding) can help defend a diagnosis. Negative findings help us "rule out" other diagnoses, or move other diagnoses down on our list. For example, consider a case of a 60-year-old man complaining of bloody stools:

Working differential: diverticulosis, colon cancer, hemorrhoids, anal fissure, angiodysplasia, inflammatory bowel disease, and ischemic colitis.

After the history and physical, you determine the no. 1 diagnosis is hemorrhoids.

1. Hemorrhoids

    History findings:

    - blood on the toilet paper after a bowel movement (positive finding)
    - hx of constipation (positive finding)
    - denies hx of weight loss (negative finding)
    - denies family hx of colon cancer (negative finding)

    Physical exam findings:

    - abdomen not tender (negative finding)
    - no masses palpated (negative finding)

Myth # 77
"I should make up findings to support my diagnosis."

Debunking the myth:
You should never fabricate positive or negative findings to support your diagnosis. If you didn't obtain the information while you were in the room, then you can't use it.

Myth # 78
"For each diagnosis, I need to list at least five History Findings and five Physical Exam Findings."

Debunking the myth:
There is no magic number for the history and physical exam findings to support the diagnosis. Depending on the case, you may have as little as one or as many as eight findings. Simply list the findings you obtained during the encounter.

11

Diagnostic Studies

Myth # 79

"I can always place physical exam maneuvers in the diagnostic studies section of the patient note, in case I run out of time."

Debunking the myth:

Only the restricted physical exam maneuvers (rectal, pelvic, genitourinary, inguinal hernia, female breast, corneal reflex examinations, or throat swab) can be listed in the diagnostic studies section of the patient note. Do not list maneuvers that you would have done if you had more time. You will waste precious note-writing time!

Myth # 80
"I need to put the diagnostic studies in order of importance."

Debunking the myth:
Unlike your list of diagnoses, you do not have to list the diagnostic studies in order of importance. Hooray! Just list the tests you want to order as fast as you can. You can list up to eight. Don't forget to list a restricted physical exam maneuver, if it was indicated.

Myth # 81

"To get the most points, I will always need to list eight diagnostic studies for each case."

Debunking the myth:

Diagnostic studies are obtained to provide information that aids in the making of a diagnosis. You should only list the tests, studies, procedures, and/or restricted physical exam maneuvers that will help you confirm the diagnosis. Listing extra studies will not give you extra points.

Myth # 82
"Every case needs diagnostic studies."

Debunking the myth:
There are cases that do not require diagnostic studies to confirm the diagnosis. If no diagnostic studies are necessary, you should write "No studies indicated." *Do not leave the section blank.*

Myth # 83
"I need to order a CBC on every case."

Debunking the myth:

I know that popular review courses encourage examinees to order common tests, like CBCs, on every case. This is ridiculous advice. Once again, you will be wasting precious note-writing time. Only order a diagnostic test if it helps you answer one question: "Will this "test" help me confirm the diagnosis?" If the answer is "yes," then include it on your list.

Myth # 84
"If a patient clearly needs an antibiotic, I should list it under the diagnostic studies."

Debunking the myth:
Although the treatment may be obvious, you will never list treatment options anywhere in the patient note.

Myth # 85

"If I believe the patient has cancer, I will refer them to an oncologist."

Debunking the myth:

You will never refer any of your patients to a specialist during the Step 2 CS exam. For this exam, imagine yourself working in a setting where you are the only provider available.

SEP Myths

12

Pronunciation

Myth # 86

"My English is horrible, but I have friends who passed and their English is worse than mine."

Debunking the myth:

Effective communication and appropriate interpersonal skills are necessary to provide quality medical care. The Step 2 CS exam is evaluating your ability to communicate effectively with patients. The standardized patients are using rating scales to assess the effort required to understand your English. If you frequently use wrong words or pronunciations, it will adversely impact your Spoken English Proficiency (SEP) score. Feeling comfortable with conversational English is fundamental to passing the USMLE Step 2 CS.

Myth # 87
"If I have an accent, I will never pass the SEP component."

Debunking the myth:
Most people who live in the United States have an accent! Take a visit to the deep south or the east coast, and you'll see what I mean! (No offence intended.) The standardized patients are familiar with accents. If you have an accent, stop worrying about it. You need to focus on the correct and appropriate use of the English language to effectively communicate with your patient.

Myth # 88

"The USMLE wants to screen out doctors who have an accent."

Debunking the myth:

The USMLE is not using the Step 2 CS exam as a screening tool to exclude doctors with accents. Speaking with an accent has no bearing on your abilities as a doctor nor need it affect your ability to understand or be understood. Many of the current practicing physicians in the United States have accents.

13

Word Choice

Myth # 89
"Using the wrong pronouns happens sometimes, but it's not a significant slip up."

Debunking the myth:

Consistently referring to someone with the wrong gender pronoun (he vs. she, him vs. her) is one of the more obvious and recognizable mistakes you can make. This frequently occurs during the telephone encounters. While questioning the caretaker about the 5-year-old girl complaining of abdominal pain, you may ask, "How long has *he* had the pain?" The caretaker will not know who you are referring to because the patient is a girl, not a boy. This will lead to confusion and ultimately frustration.

English has gender-specific pronouns. If you have trouble with them, practice!

Myth # 90

"It's a waste of my time learning common words and phrases people use to describe their medical condition and symptoms."

Debunking the myth:

The patients aren't going to describe their complaints using medical terms. They are going to use words, expressions, or phrases that someone who has no medical knowledge would use. In order for you to understand them, you'll need to know these terms. If you feel this may be an issue, you need to supplement your preparation for this exam. Practice using commonly used words in place of the medical terms. Some examples are as follows: pass out versus syncope, pain with urination versus dysuria, short of breath versus dyspnea, double vision versus diplopia. Refer to http://www.nlm.nih.gov/medlineplus/mplusdictionary.html for more suggestions.

Myth # 91
"If the patient uses a slang word that I don't understand, I should just pretend like I do."

Debunking the myth:
"I've been barfing all day!" This was the chief complaint of my husband's first patient in the United States. He went to medical school in Italy and had just arrived to start his internal medicine residency. He had no idea what she meant.

If your patient uses a word you are unfamiliar with, ask them to clarify the meaning. "Tell me exactly what you mean by barfing." (FYI, it's slang for vomiting.) Never pretend to understand a word that you don't understand. It will ultimately hurt your SEP and CIS score.

Miscellaneous Myths

14

Things to Remember

Myth # 92
"I read on a forum...."

Debunking the myth:

Don't read any forums! And after you take the exam, don't share any information about your cases. You should never share or read any information about the Step 2 CS cases! The USMLE has a policy prohibiting this behavior. Please refer to the "Testing Regulations and Rules of Conduct" in the CS Content Description and General Information pdf (cs-info-manual.pdf).

Myth # 93
"Once I register for the exam, I do not have to refer back to the USMLE website."

Debunking the myth:
Occasionally, the USMLE policies change. When this occurs, they post the information on the USMLE website. The announcement for the change will be on the home page: http://www.usmle.org/. I recommend that you check the website weekly once you register for any of the USMLE exams.

Myth # 94

"If I score high on one of the subcomponents, it will pull up one of my weaker scores and I'll still pass."

Debunking the myth:

The Step 2 CS exam is unique from the other USMLE exams because it is not scored as one exam. You'll be scored on the three separate subcomponents: Integrated Clinical Encounter, Communication and Interpersonal Skills, and Spoken English Proficiency. Each of the three subcomponents is independent of each other and must be passed on the same day in order for you to achieve a passing performance on the exam. What this means is that you could perform perfectly on two of the three subcomponents, but if you fail one, you fail the exam.

Myth # 95
"The cases are impossible to do in 15 minutes."

Debunking the myth:
Each case is created for a 15-minute scenario. The USMLE does not create complicated cases that can't be solved within 15 minutes. If you use your medical knowledge and diagnostic reasoning skills to ask pertinent questions and perform a focused physical exam, you will be able to collect enough information to develop a differential diagnosis and an initial diagnostic plan.

Myth # 96
"The USMLE uses the videotapes to score me."

Debunking the myth:
The videotapes are not used for the initial scoring of your exam. The USMLE has determined that standardized patients capture your communication skills better than a third person observing a video tape. The videos are used for quality control and research purposes.

Myth # 97
"Checking my watch will help me keep track of the time during each encounter."

Debunking the myth:
You are not allowed to wear a watch during the exam. There is a clock in each room to help you manage the time. Also, there will be an announcement when there are five minutes remaining in each encounter.

Myth # 98
"I plan on bringing my lucky pen."

Debunking the myth:
You cannot use your "lucky pen" during the exam. The USMLE will give you a standard-issue pen. In addition, you should not bring a cell phone, pager, or study notes. There will be a place to store your personal items during the exam.

Myth # 99
"Only 10 of the 12 cases are scored."

Debunking the myth:
The Step 2 CS exam includes 12 patient encounters. There are a very small number of pilot cases, which are unscored. However, you'll never know which cases are pilots. Therefore, assume you are getting scored on all 12 of your cases.

Myth # 100
"I use an inhaler for my asthma; therefore, I can bring it to the test center."

Debunking the myth:

Before your examination day, you need to submit a written request for the use of any medications, external appliances, or electronic devices. Examples include medications, insulin pumps, syringes, inhalers, breast pumps, crutches, casts, wheelchairs, and hearing aids.

Myth # 101
"I need to bring only my Scheduling Permit and an unexpired ID."

Debunking the myth:
You need to bring the following:

1. Scheduling Permit

2. Confirmation notice

3. Unexpired government-issued photo ID

4. Standard stethoscope

5. White lab coat

*and … y*our common sense.

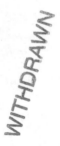